Sex...

A Spiritual Guide

for the youth of today

By Nan Sea

For ordering information
call 1(800) 822-1197

or write:
Spirit Script
P.O. Box 1374
Summit, N.J. 07902-1374

Copyright © 1995 by Nancy Seabold

All rights reserved,
including the right of reproduction
in whole or in part in any form.
For permission please write
or call the publisher.

Library of Congress
Catalogue Card Number: 94-93913

ISBN 0-9643852-0-1

I am neither a psychologist, nor an authority on human sexuality. I offer my thoughtful consideration as a mother of two daughters, and as a spiritual person on a path toward my own discovery. Inspiration for this book came to me out of the process of *journeying. Such inspiration is sacred to me, so I have treated it in that way, quite literally as received.

*Journeying is a spiritual method used to gain wisdom. Like meditation, it helps one to find the "heart" of issues, to reach beyond the psychological and intellectual dimensions.

Each of us has the human potential to tap into the higher voice from within ourselves and to reach out for answers. We may pray to God. We may seek infinite wisdom from the "spirit voice" with meditation or journeying.

How you define God and your spirituality is dependent upon the influence of your family's religious heritage and the development of your own spiritual philosophy along side or apart from that tradition. One needs time to read and to ponder in order to develop a personal spiritual philosophy. What is crucial, however is finding the connection with one's own spiritual self in order to more clearly find answers to important questions.

It may also be helpful to discuss key issues with people you respect who know you well, such as parents, counselors, or a friend whose judgement you value. Questions regarding sexuality are among the most difficult to address. Some answers can only be found in quiet reflection. You may want to look at issues such as: How can one deal with the natural pull between one's inherent sexuality and timing... As in waiting for the right relationship... Or if you have found that relationship... Waiting for the appropriate time to become involved?

It is unrealistic to deny the presence of our sexuality. It is a natural part of being human. But other areas of compatibility can be explored first. With regards to physical compatibility, affection can be mutually communicated without completion of the act, for example.

It can be a challenge to wait if you feel you are in love. Feeling "in love" however, might not mean you are completely decided on all facets of the relationship. If you do consummate the relationship before being completely committed, it can become confusing. If sex is compelling and satisfying, you may not be completely honest with yourself regarding the other facets of your relationship.

Perspective may be blurred by the need to have the physical connection. Pain is involved in separation. If things do not work out, you may suffer emotionally, mentally, spiritually, or physically.

When the sexual relationship is of spirit, sex is reflective of the stage that you are at with your partner. It stays at the appropriate level. This level is defined by the degree of genuine love you feel; love affected by the discovery of other attributes besides just physical attraction. Sex of the spirit is able to wait for that exploration and discovery.

Just as it is easy and appropriate to give a kiss on the cheek or a big bear hug to a friend for example... When you are in touch with spirit, it is then easy to *walk* through the stages of love. Sex is a beautiful part of life. Being honest with sexual expression honors the spirit.

With spirit honored, sexual involvement becomes a result of feelings, not the reverse. Feelings that come as a result of putting the act first or sexual expression too early are not only confusing, but misrepresentative of who you are as a holistic person... A person of body, mind, *and* spirit.

When spirit is a part of our lives, it actively affects our actions. When one has walked through the steps of expressing sexuality in a growing relationship, the intensity of pleasure heightens. When sex is placed in the context of true love and commitment, the highest level of personal fulfillment is reached. The degree of sacredness one attaches to sex relates directly to the level of fulfillment we receive in return.

When you are ready for commitment and when all is connected in a holistic fashion, love-making can be sacred and powerful, taking on meaning far beyond physical satisfaction.

When one is totally committed, one is first and foremost "married" in heart and spirit. Formal marriage is a perfect ideal. But if that marriage is primarily one of convenience, or if it is one without mutual heart and spirit, it will be empty and can not satisfy.   So look for commitment of the heart and spirit first. They are most important of all.

    Learning about oneself spiritually is the best thing one can do before acting. One will then have the reward of making decisions that positively affect our personal relationships and life in general.

> Love is union with somebody,
> or something, outside oneself,
> under the condition of retaining
> the separateness and integrity
> of one's own self.
> Erich Fromm, "The Sane Society"

    Evaluating and understanding relationship is something single people of all ages have struggled with. With older people, life experience may help, but sometimes that is gleaned from painful misjudgments. Then, one must heal in order to genuinely love again.

The youth of today has a struggle also, often dealing with an enormous range of opinions, some in direct opposition to each other, as in the voices from home and place of worship, compared to the opinion and experiences of classmates. The media often *totally* diverges, expressing stark viewpoints, in addition to reflecting the harsh realities of statistics. Film, though inspiring in many areas, bombards us with a stretch of the moral imagination, making any overstepping of our *own* boundaries tame by comparison.

It is difficult to hold on to one's spiritual center when the voices around us are so loud. Quiet is needed to hear the voice of spirit and the quiet voice from within.

Be true to your own feelings, as you walk through the stages of love. How we use our sexuality and to what degree is an enormous responsibility, affecting our own well being as well as that of our partner.

> To thine own self be true,
> And it must follow,
> as the night the day,
> Thou canst not then be false to any man.
> Shakespeare, *Hamlet* Act I, sc. 3, 78

In being true to ourselves, we will also be true to our partners. One can ponder and one can read, but best, one can take a journey deep into oneself to seek spirit... By meditating and journeying, using methods in addition to prayer that help us seek the "God" in ourselves, and the God "voice" of the Universe.

As we more clearly define our spiritual existence, relationships are enhanced. When decisions are made through the spiritual frame of reference, we wait to become involved. It is neither just because we have held on to a religious code of ethics, nor is it just because it will please our families. It is because we care about ourselves enough to want a meaningful and happy life, where deep in our souls we feel fed by our existence.

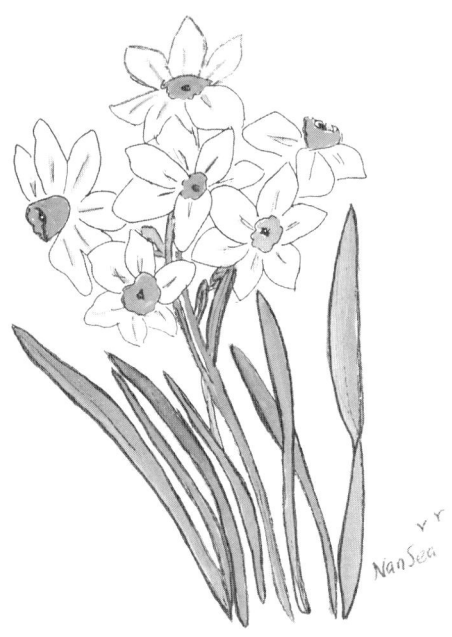

I am deeply grateful to my parents and to my family for always "being there", believing in me, and for giving me the challenge.

Long ago...
  Simple talks...
    Two sweet faces,
      whose innocent queries
        touched my heart...
  We talked about love, about marriage.

Now, watching my eldest depart for college,
  discovering so much on her own...
    May there be time for reflection.

Now, observing my youngest,
  a sophomore in high school,
    swimming her energized beat...
May she feel the pulse of spirit,
  and hear it's gentle words.

Guide them both with wisdom.
  Protect them from pain and mistakes.

Dedicated to my daughters,
*   Amy and Lauren,*
*   the love for whom*
*   inspired me*
*   to seek answers...*

*   Mom*

Reflections from a journey...

A gift to share with my daughters...
And one I now share with you.

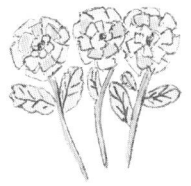

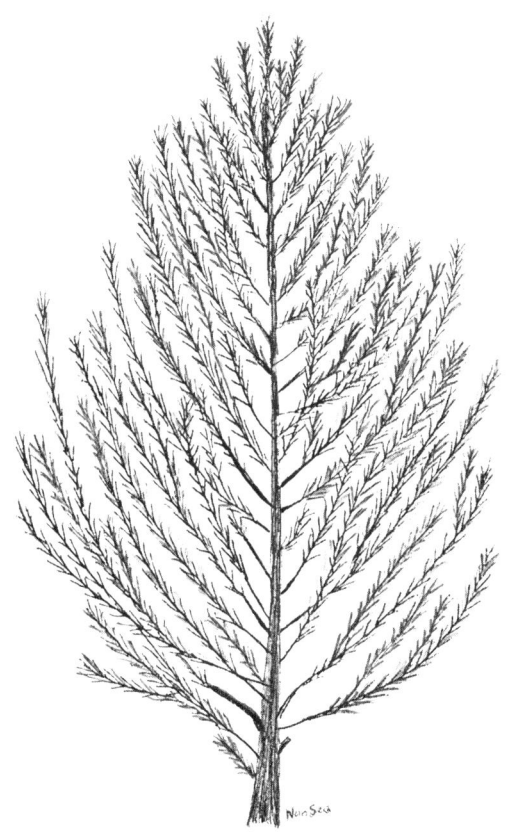

Don't get stuck
in body sensations.

As you feel your base,
move your feelings
upward

to be sure
of what you're feeling.

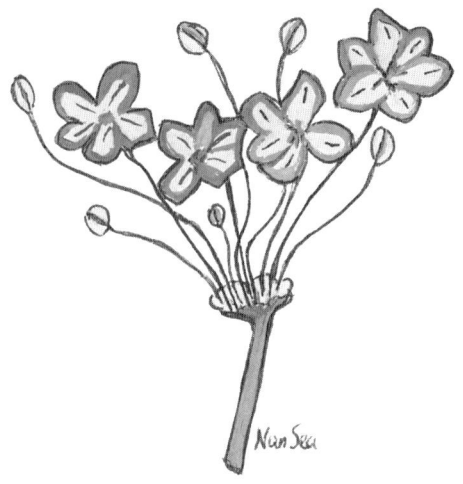

Be comfortable
with other aspects

of each other
first.

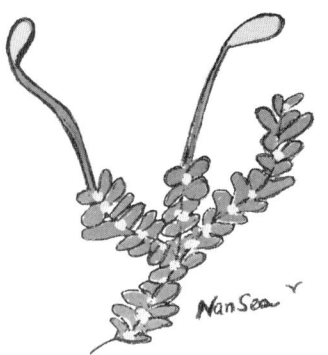

Know how to stop,

and that you can stop.

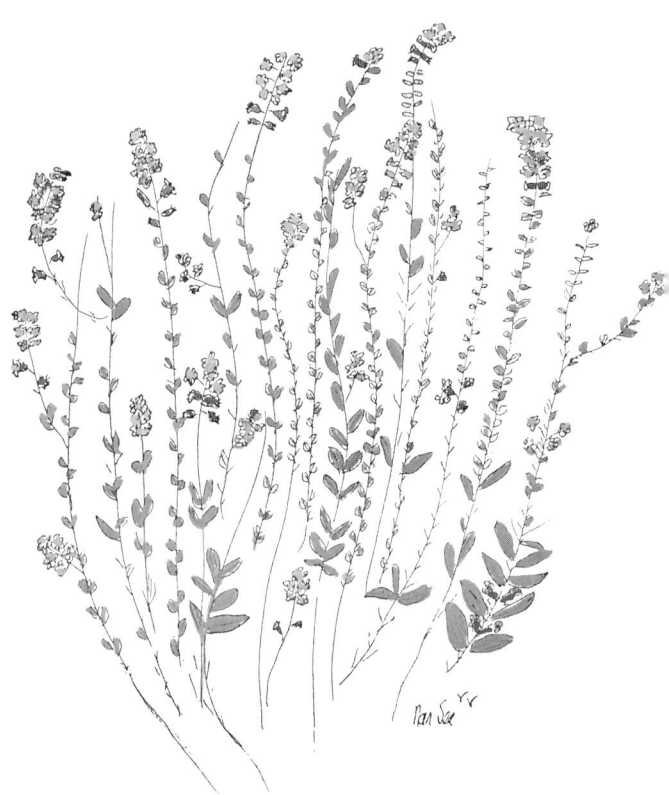

Know that it is blessed

to wait.

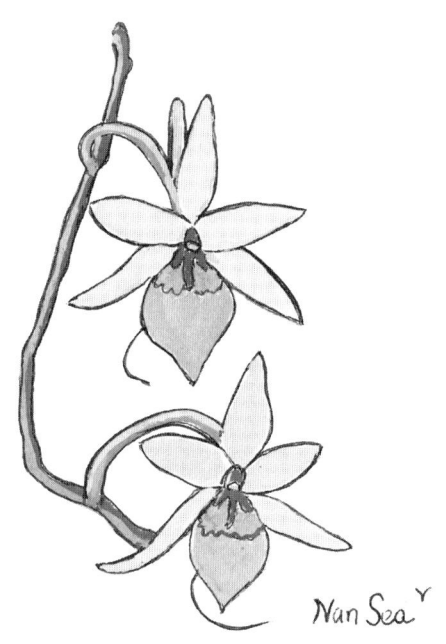

Respect
for both people's spirit
must be there,

or it takes
the dignity away
from having sex.

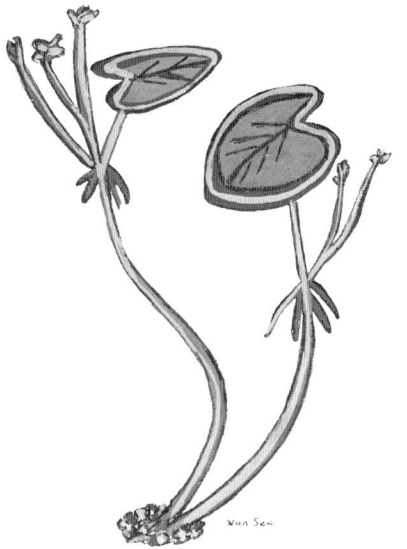

If the "upper selves"
of both people
take part
in the decision,

sex is like a blessing
or a prayer.

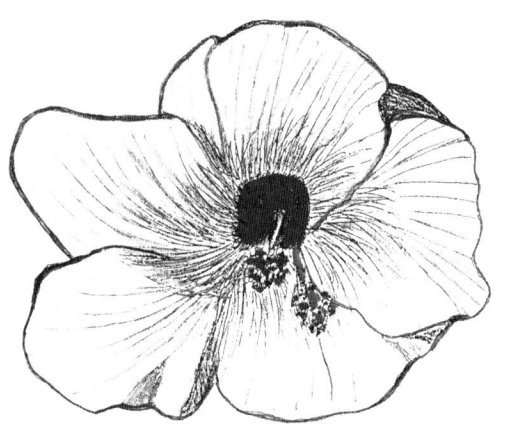

Sex is blessed

if it is made sacred.

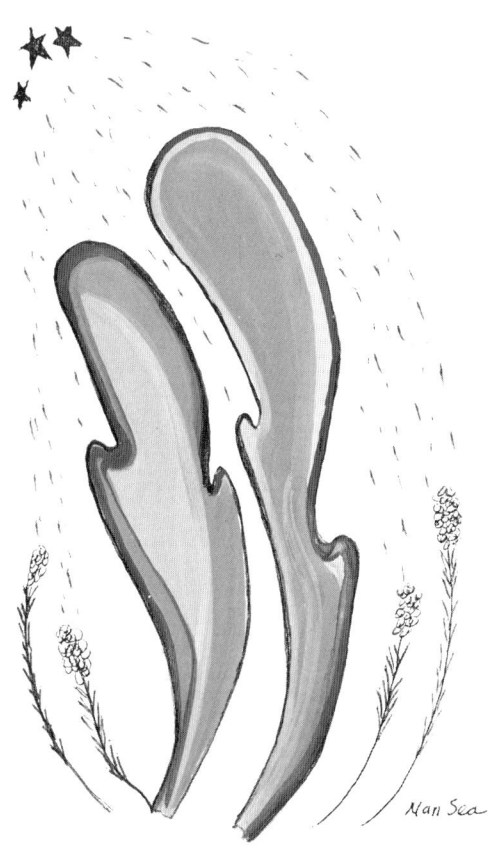

Be sure
the person
you are with
is using their heart,
mind and spirit,

and that you both
respect each other.

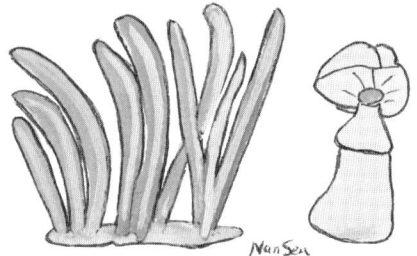

Sex
can make you
feel closer,

but at the same time
can emphasize
ways in which
you are mismatched.

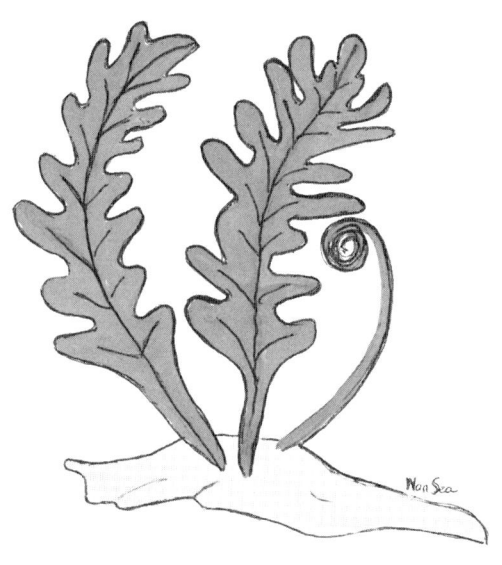

Do you care enough

to ask each other
questions?

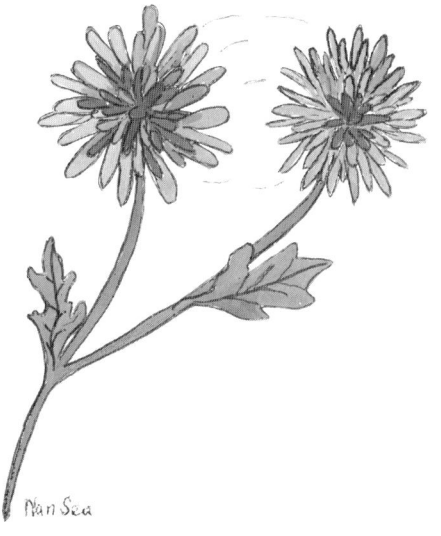

Be in touch
with your feelings

enough to share them.

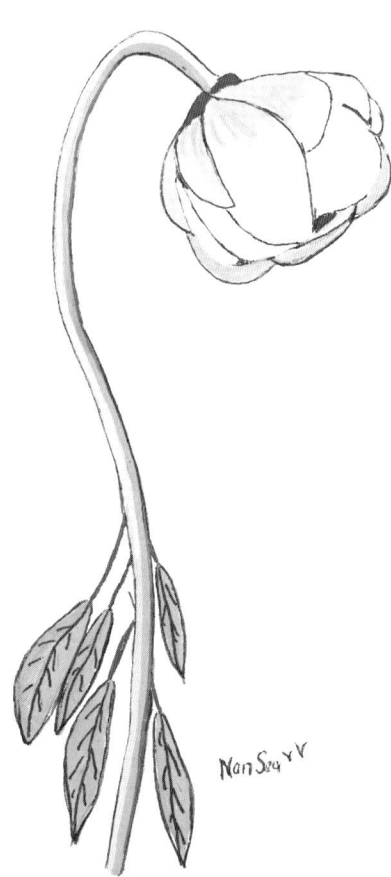

You do not want
to come away
feeling exploited,
vulnerable,
or left alone.

If you feel
any of those feelings,
you weren't in touch
with your spirit.

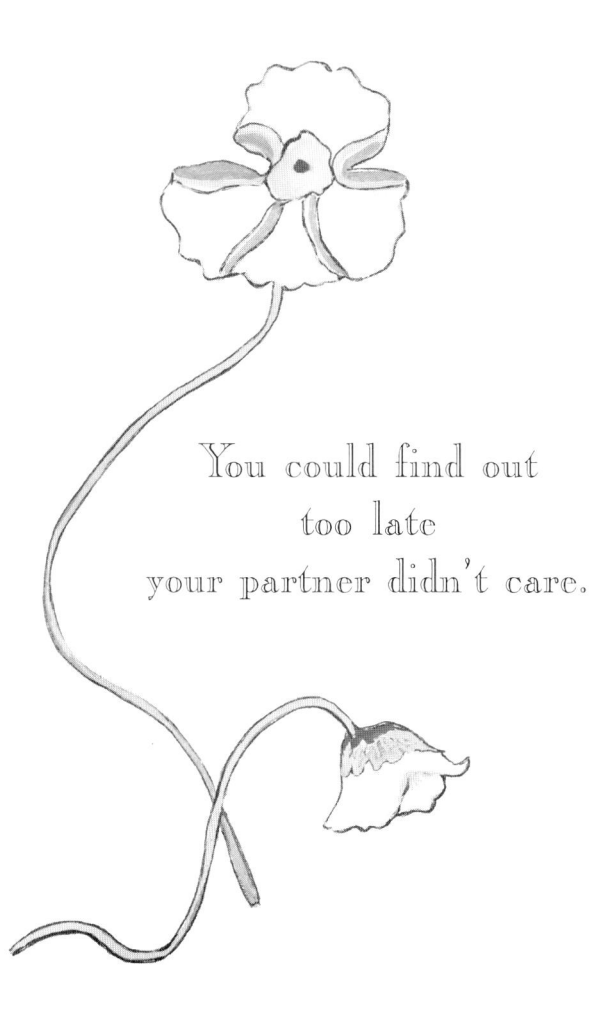

Misguided souls
would have us believe
it is enough
to lust.

Though
we do lust,

And though it is easy
to be enticed...

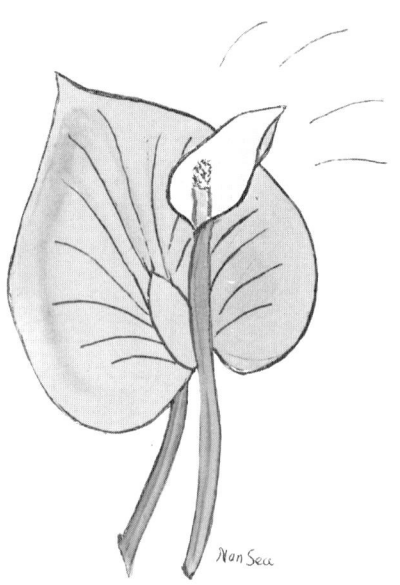

Try to put
your heart and spirit
first.

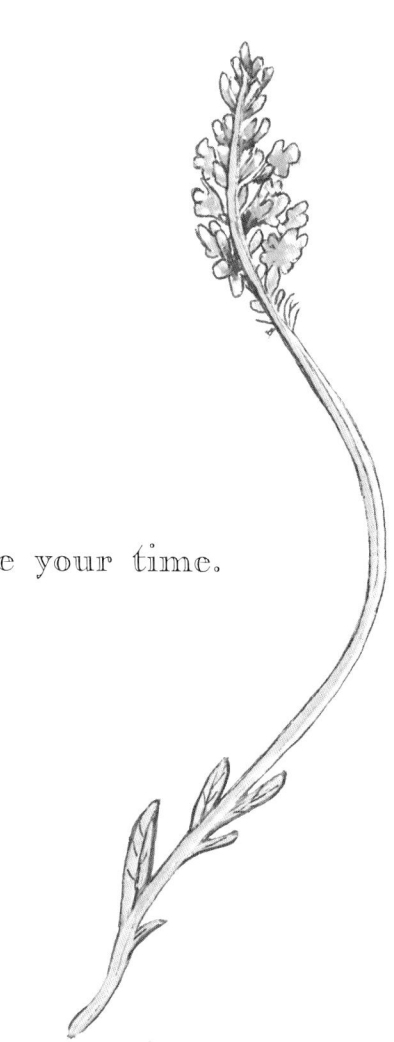

Take your time.

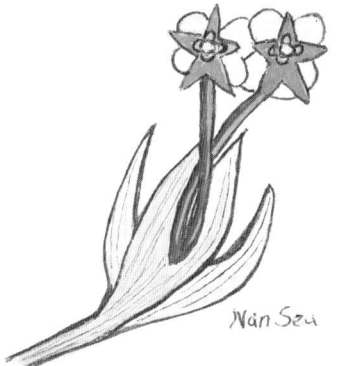

It is
the closeness of sex

that shows us how
the rest
of our relationship
should be.

If one withholds
their anger,
fear, and joy
from the other,
or if one
does not know
how to intimately
share these things,

one will feel empty.

One will be
all the more hungry
for intimacy.

Your partner
is not likely
to understand
the hunger,
as feelings
were not fully discussed.

Not understanding
each other,
the partners then feel
they can't satisfy
each other.

Both partners
become unhappy.

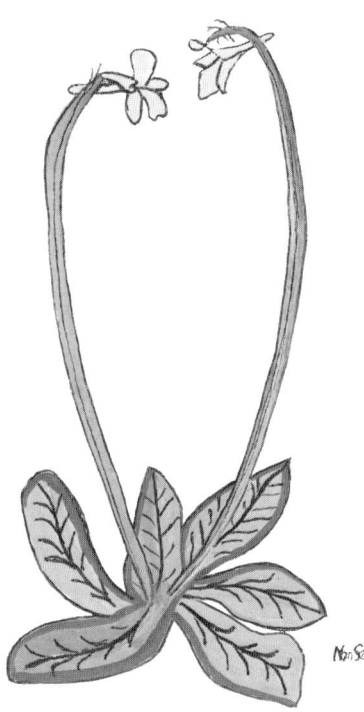

So, if there are
missing pieces

and if the partners
are unable
to work
on those pieces,

sex will feel empty.

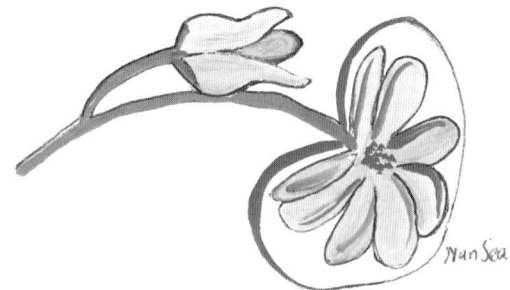

One can not have doubts
and enjoy another fully.

Something will always
be held back.

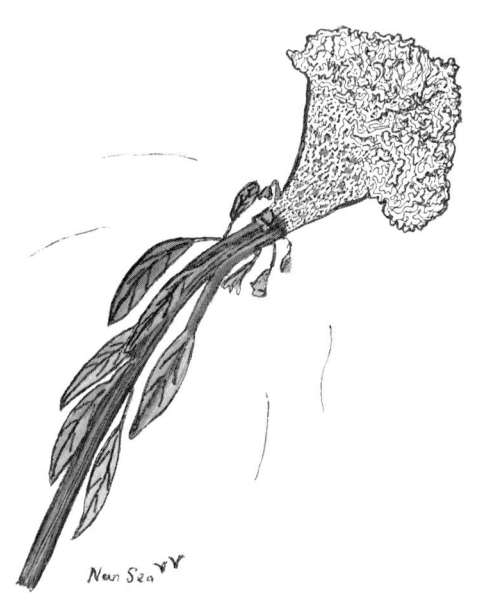

Sex
is not
to be taken lightly.

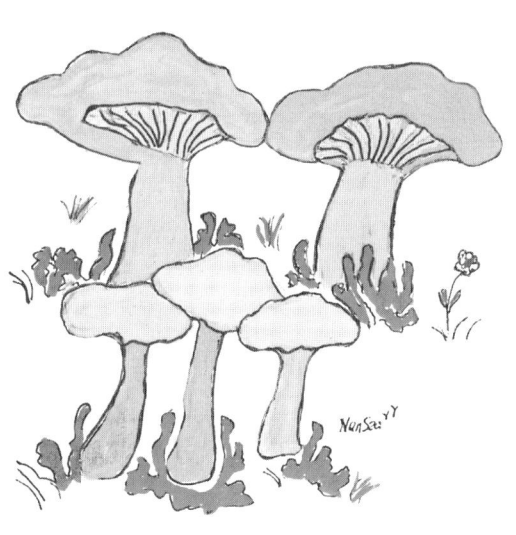

Sex can help you
stay together,

and to build
a family.

It is one
of the most sacred
vows you take
outside of the solemn vow
to each other.

If you take it lightly
and endorse yourself
with your body only,

the pain
and abandonment
will be enormous

because
you will be left
craving a body.

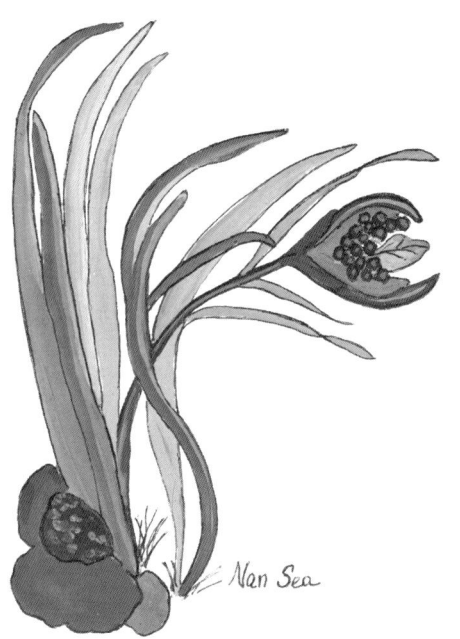

People know how
to protect themselves
against the perils of sex,

but they are naive
as to the perils of sex
on the psyche.

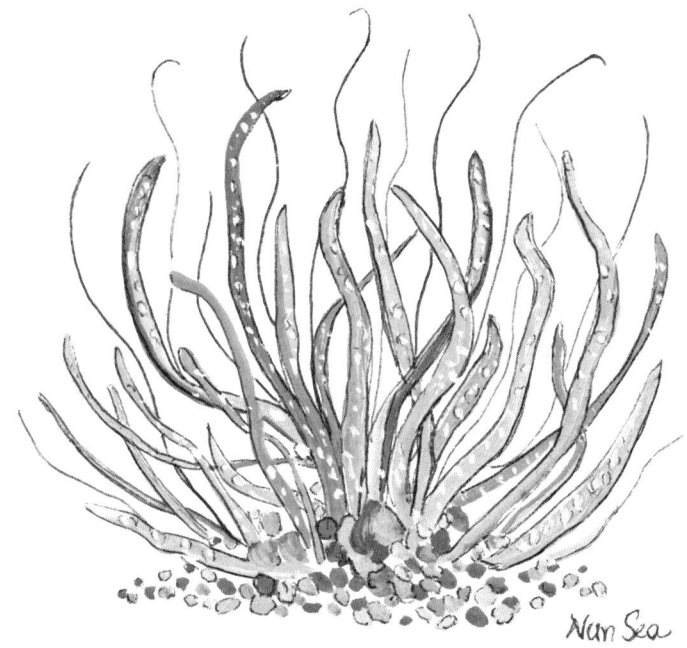

Sex
is not
for
many partners.

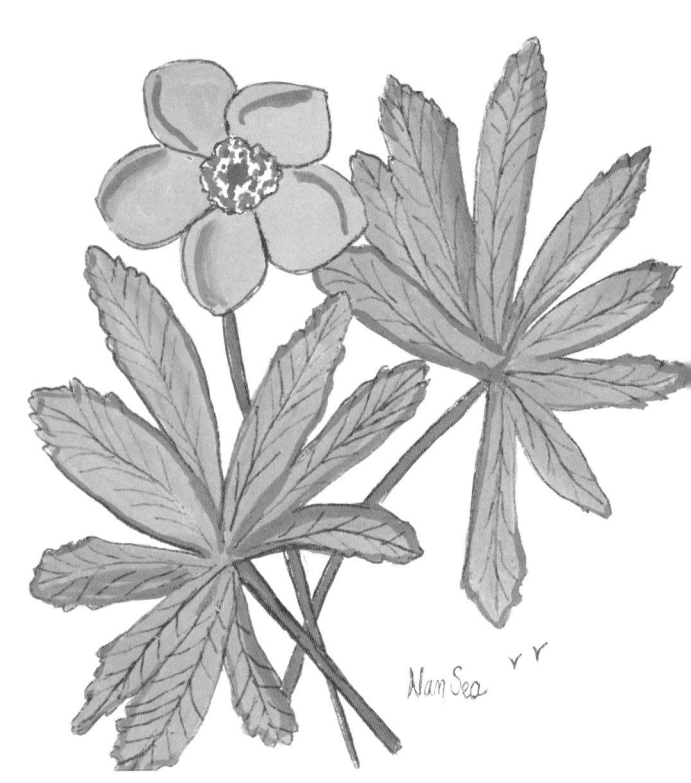

Sex
is for
a purposely chosen mate,

a partner
with whom
you can be intimate

on many different levels.

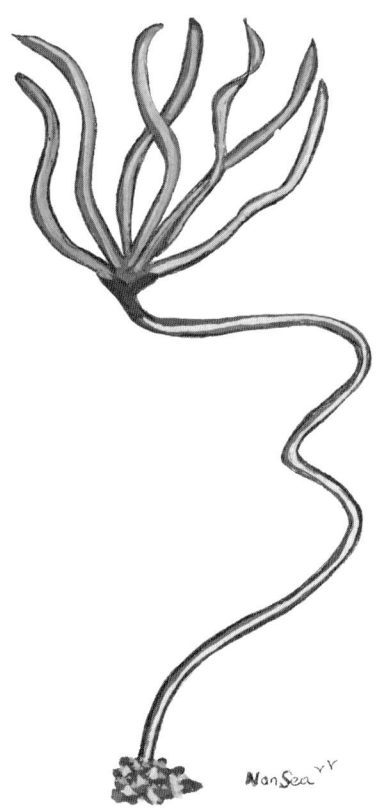

It is not
a game,

nor mindless dance.

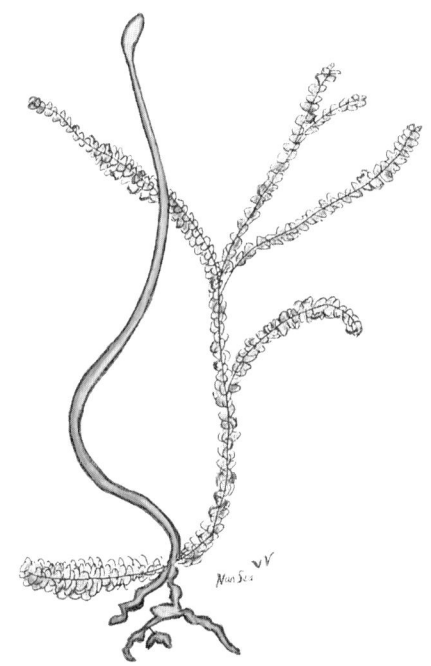

It is not
for hedonistic
thrill seekers,

though many
use it
in that way.

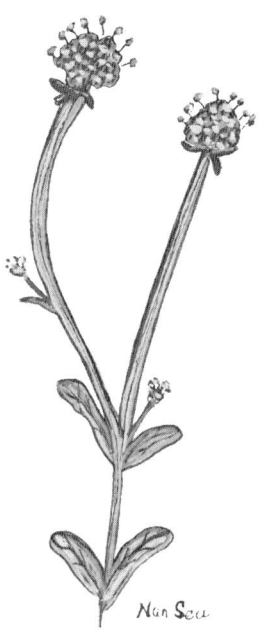

Those who fall prey
to empty bliss

are never
truly satisfied.

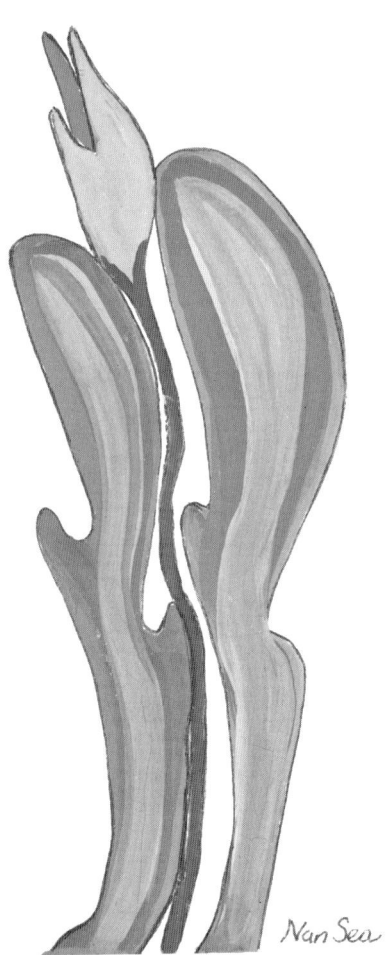

Reserve making love

for when
you treasure

all that you have
with your partner.

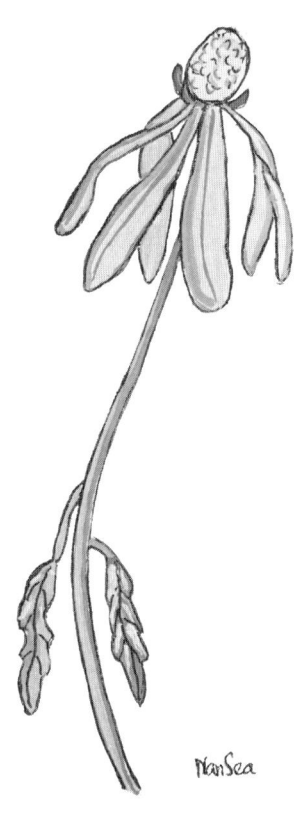

Give your body freely
without intent
of heart and mind,

and it will be valued less

until the "you" in yourself
has lost it's meaning.

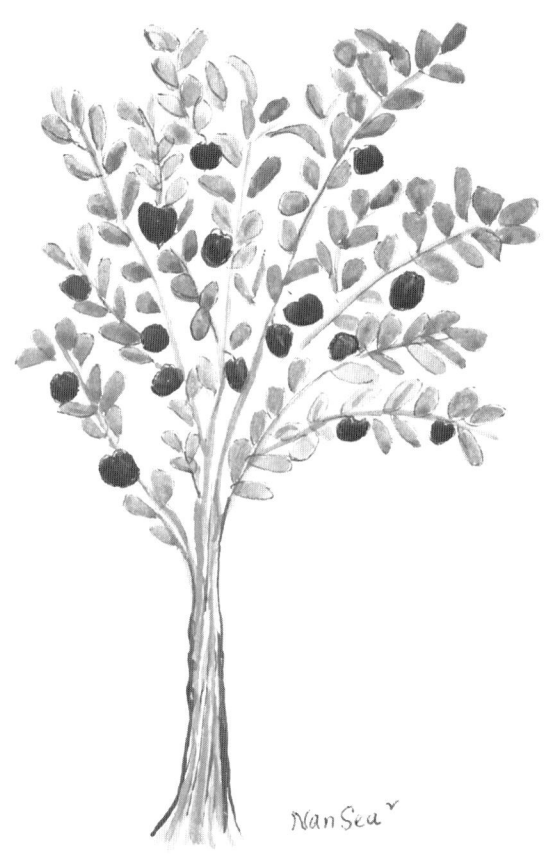

Only as long
as we take care of our bodies...

Can our goals reach fruition.

But if
you make a mistake,

it's not too late
to correct it,
for we are all human.

We all err.

The pain that mistakes create
is enough to bear.

We must move forward

and try again.

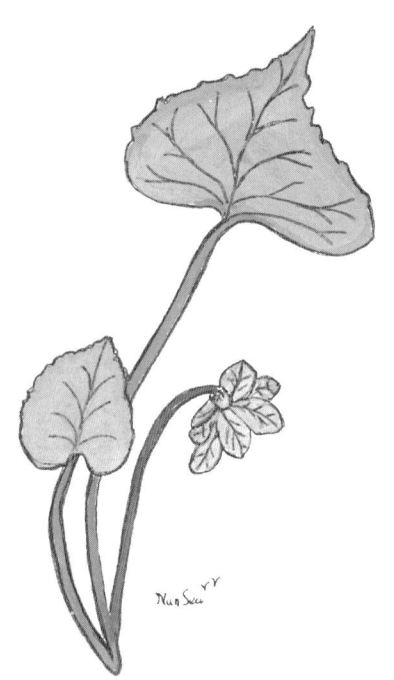

Blessed are they
who keep their heart.

They will have
a bigger heart to give.

❊ *" So we know and believe the love God has for us.
God is love, and he who abides in love
abides in God, and God abides in him."
(The Bible: I John 4:16)*

*"There is no fear in love, but perfect love
casts out fear. For fear has to do
with punishment, and he who fears
is not perfected in love."
(The Bible: I John 4:18)*

❊ ❊ *However you personally define God...
The Divine, Universal, Infinite source*

We often
separate ourselves
from our hearts,

but we must never
stop striving
for *perfect love
as * *God has taught us.

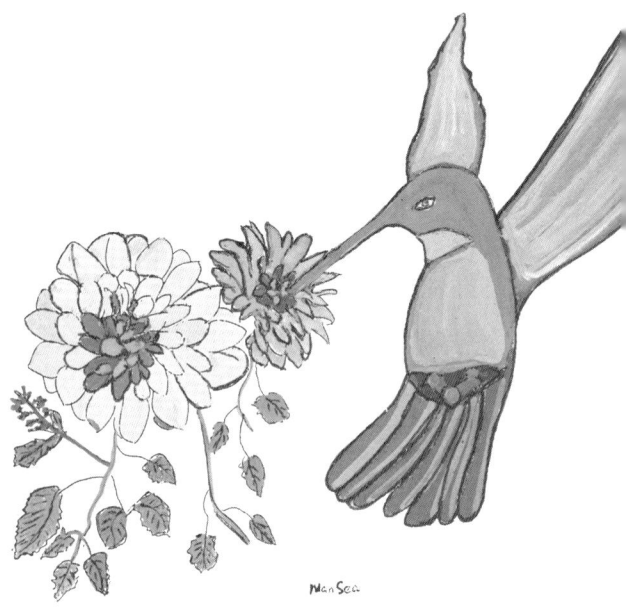

We as children of God
can only try,

but it is in trying
that we are most justly
rewarded.

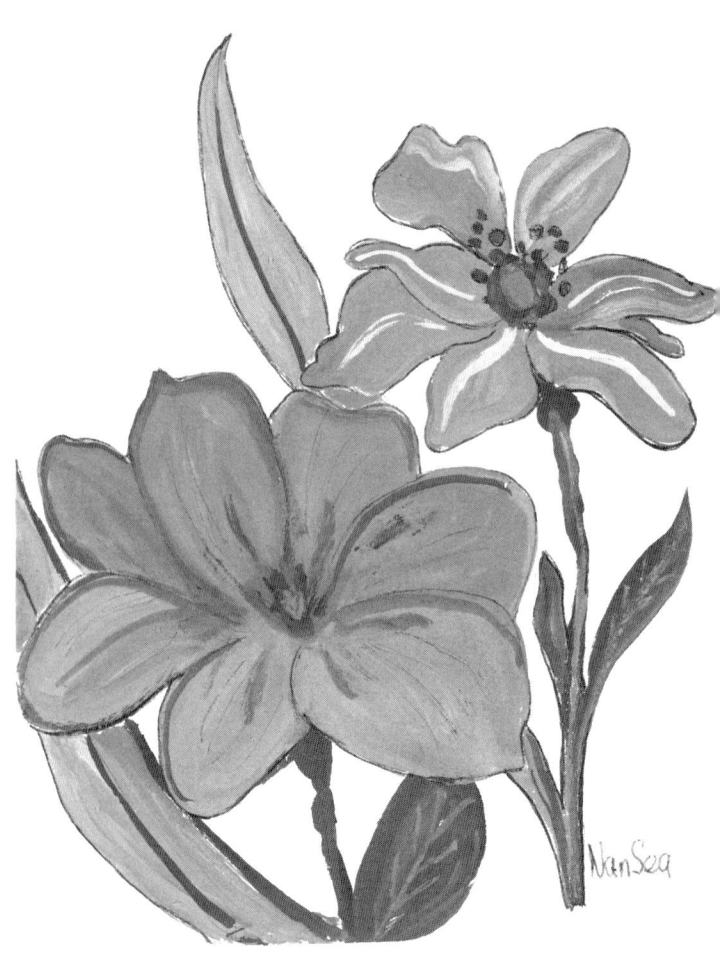

Keep your heart
pure and innocent.

You will attract good
and will be rewarded
accordingly.

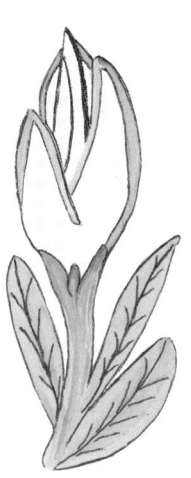

As the level
of communication
increases,

so too will your
level of intimacy.

When there is true love
and open communication...
When two people
are working in harmony
toward love
and completeness...
When those people
are being all they can be
as individuals
and as a couple,
and then
give their bodies freely...

Those partners
will have
a binding physical union
that seals the vow
to each other,

by the very commitment
of trying hard,
and fully
enjoying each other.

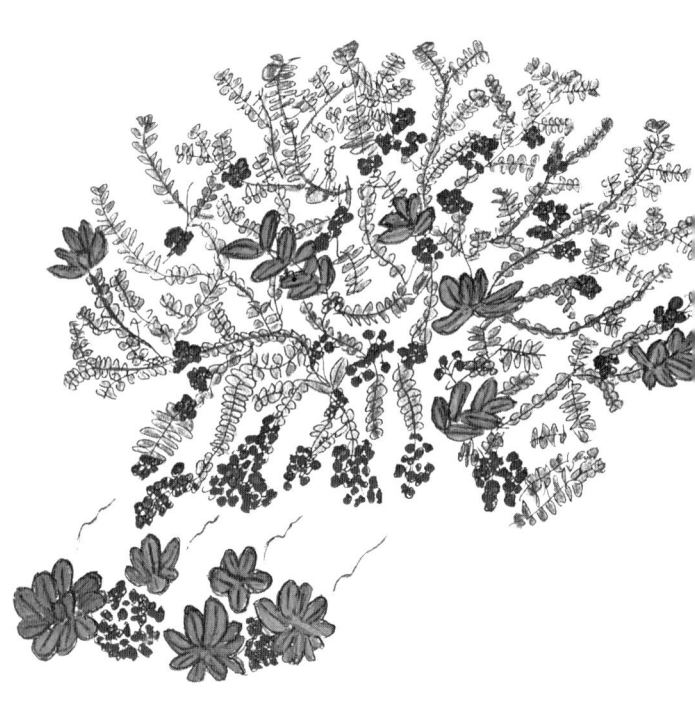

That couple
and each
of those two people
individually,

can add even more fully
to the community,
to the earth,
and to the universe.

God gives us one body,

and one body
can be so easily
trampled on.

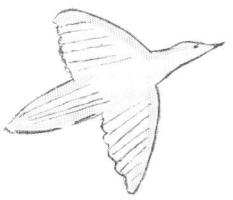

God gives us one soul,
so that it
can be raised

and fly with joy.

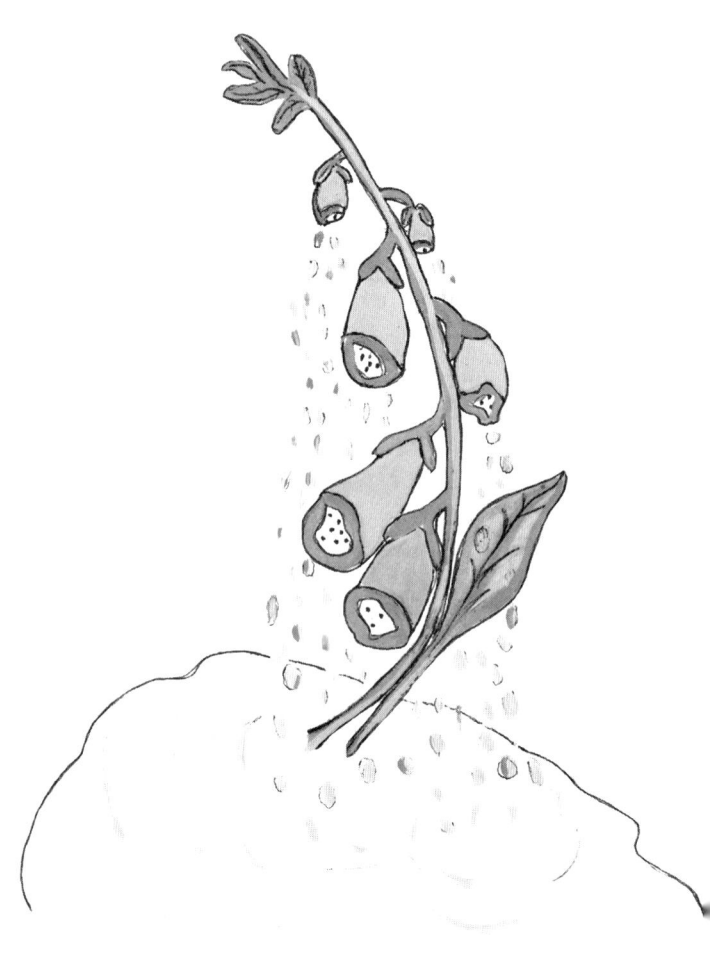

The universe weeps
at frivolous love.

If you give your body
to many,

it will be treasured not.

But if you wait
you will be rewarded.

For when the time
is right,

you will know
it is right.

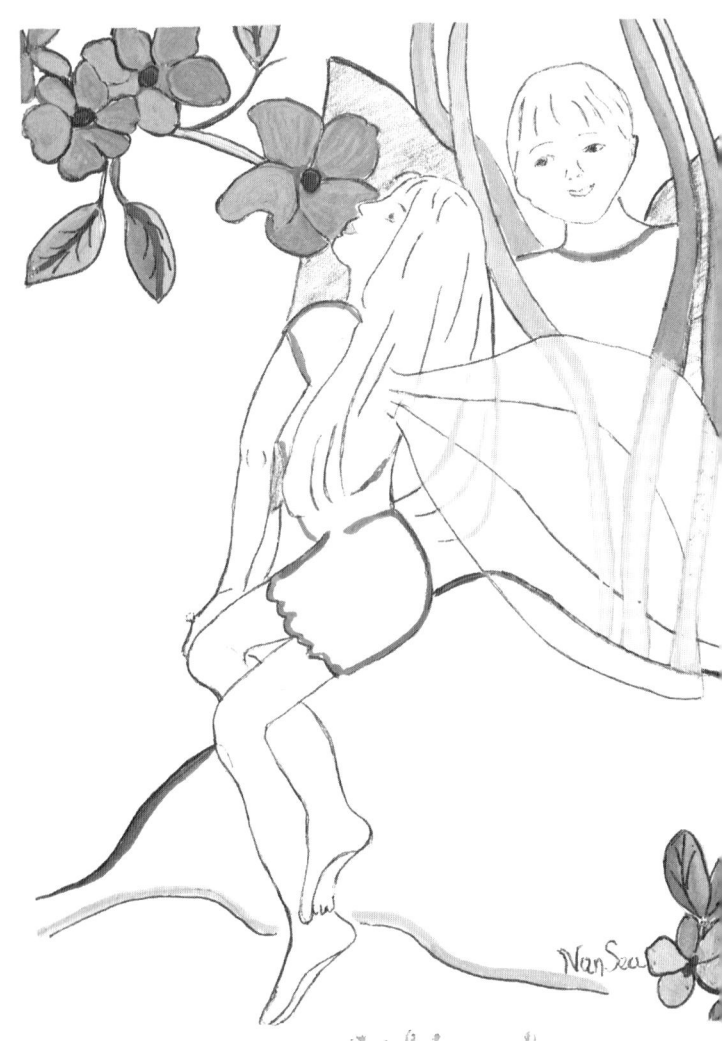

Sex can be
as playful
as innocent children,

yet as pure
as awakening spirit.

*"Do you not know that
your body is a temple
of the Holy Spirit
within you,
which you have
from God?..."*

The Bible, I Corinthians, 6:19

※ Our body
is our temple,

to be treated
with respect.

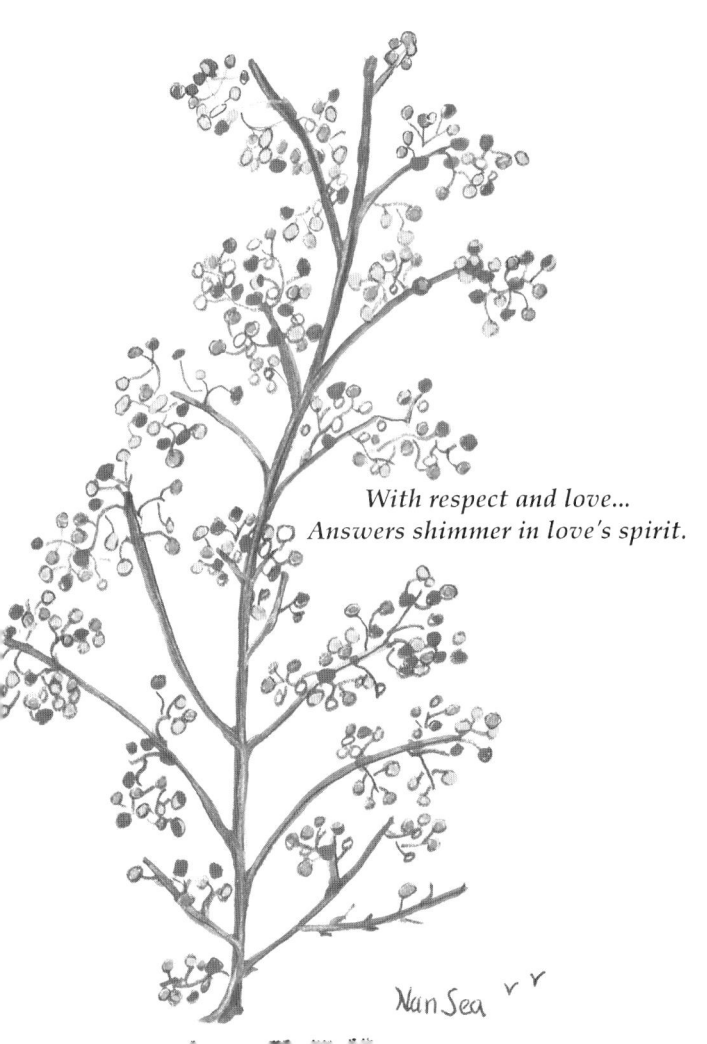

With respect and love...
Answers shimmer in love's spirit.

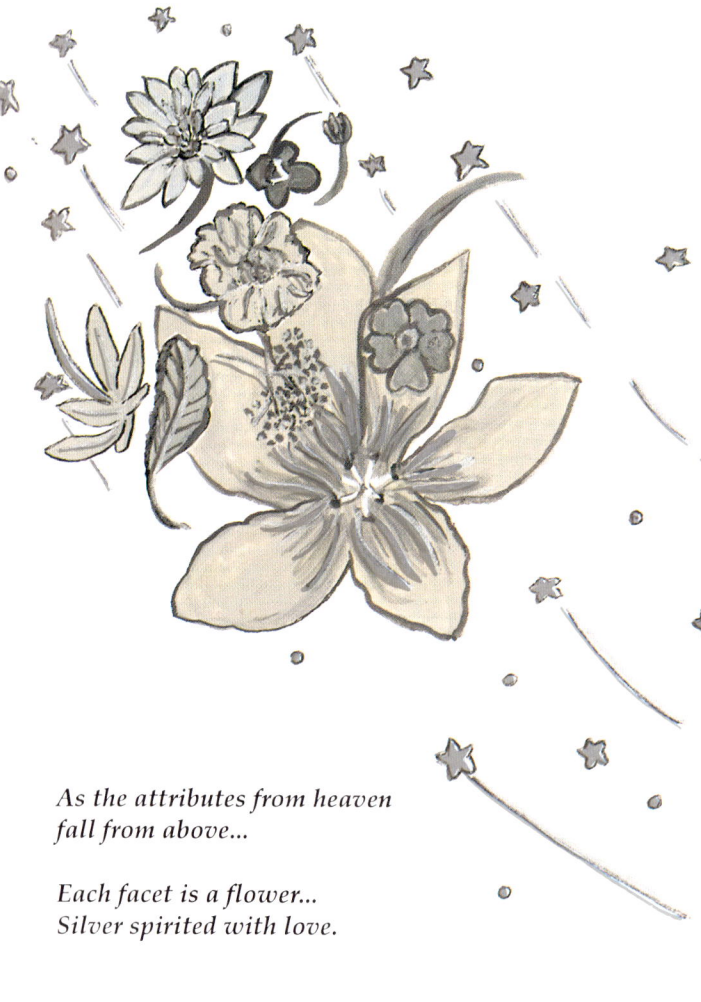

*As the attributes from heaven
fall from above...*

*Each facet is a flower...
Silver spirited with love.*

When
the many facets of love
are there...
When committed
to each other...
Do not be ashamed
to enjoy each other fully.
Physical love
will nourish
the relationship.

Falling from God's hearts to ours...

Spirit

Heart   Knowledge

Patience

Respect   Sensitivity

Intimacy

Communication

Desire & Ability to Grow

Commitment

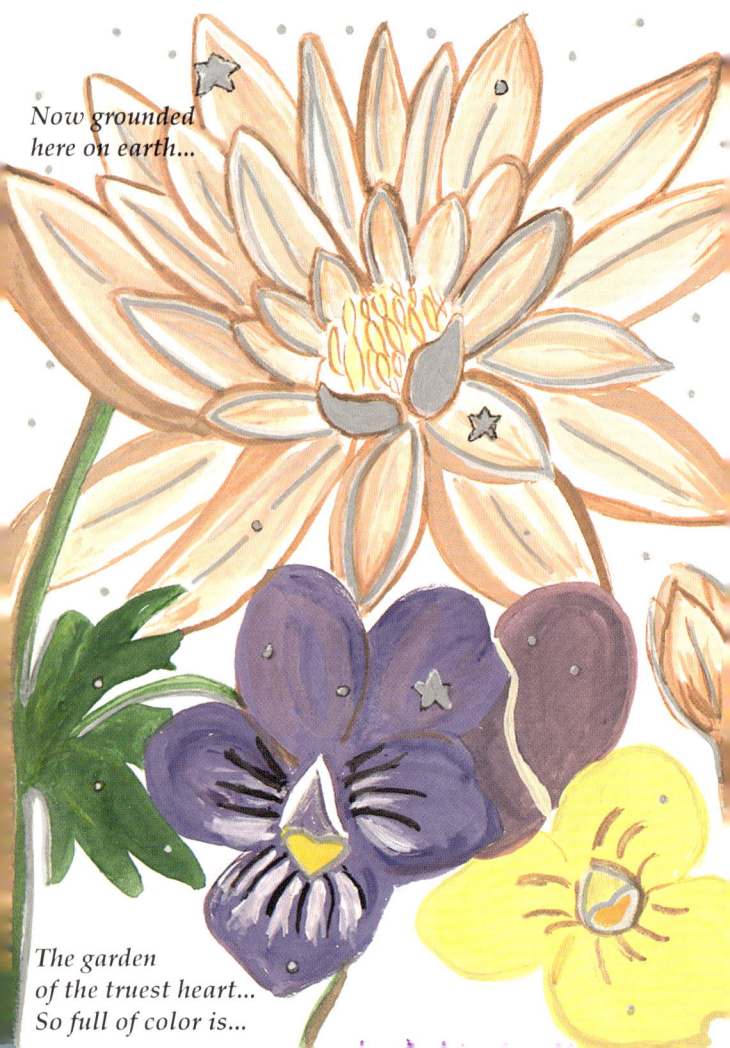

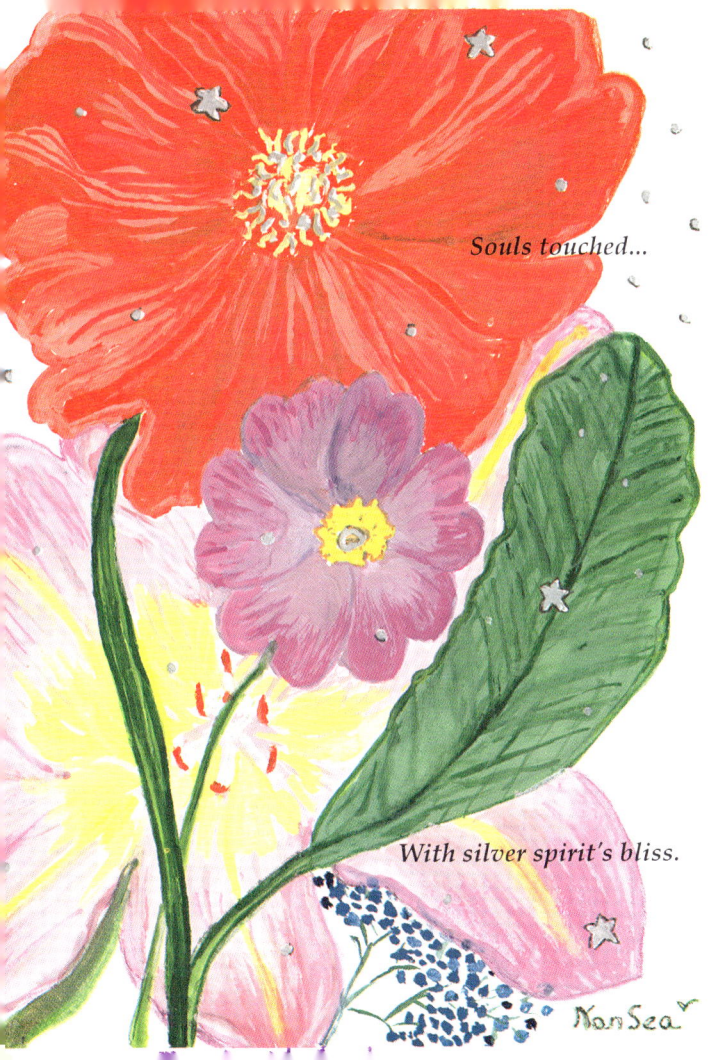

Spirit of all Divine...

*Make more clear
the attributes of spirit.*

*Fall from the heavens
into my heart...*

So I may once again remember...

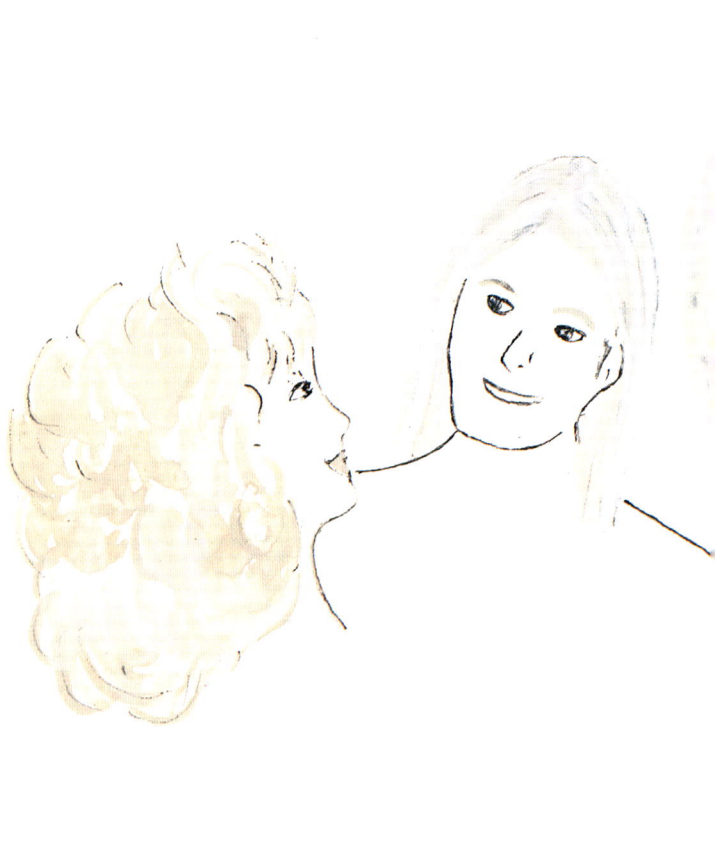

We must first recognize
love in ourselves...

So that
we may see it
in another.

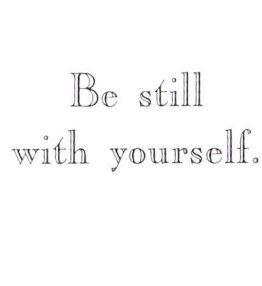

Be still
with yourself.

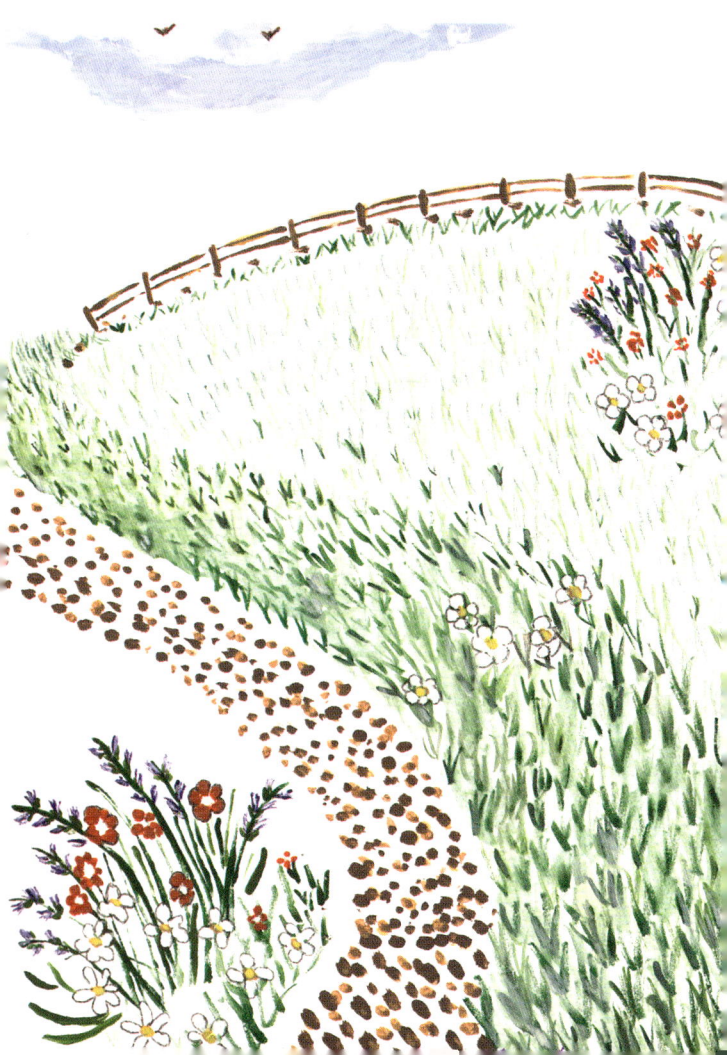

*May those searching
for love's communion
reach up,
reach inward, as well.*

*May you find love
in your happiness.*

Nan Sea

Soon to follow...
"After the Commitment"...

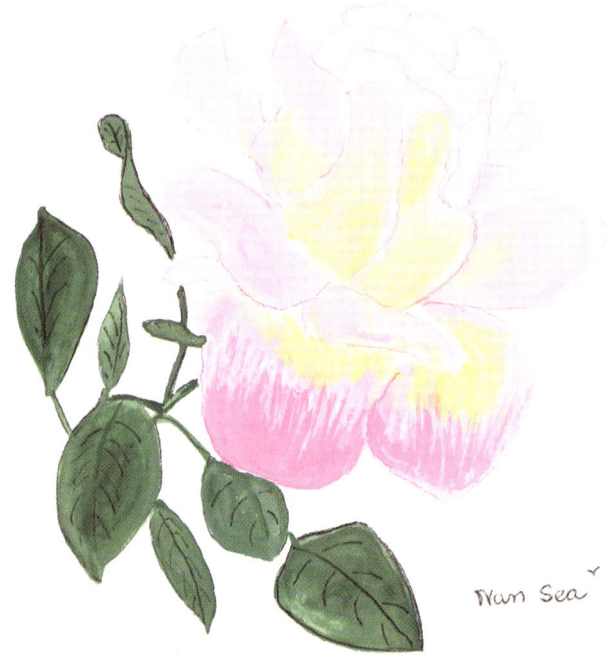

A small gift book
by Nan Sea.

To order copies of
"Sex... A Spiritual Guide"
send $9.95.
(N.J. residents add $.60 sales tax.)

Mailing:
Please add $1.50 per book.

Send check or money order to:
Spirit Script
P.O. Box 1374
Summit, N.J. 07902-1374

Name:_____
Address:_____
City:_____
State:_____ Zip:_____
Phone:_____